NCCN Guidelines for Patients®

The essential guide for people facing cancer.

Based on care recommendations from leading cancer experts.

Explains high-quality cancer care provided at state-of-the-art cancer centers.

Reviewed and revised every year.

Did you know that top cancer centers across the United States work together to improve cancer care? This alliance of leading cancer centers is called the National Comprehensive Cancer Network® (NCCN®).

Because cancer care is always evolving, NCCN develops and frequently updates evidence-based cancer care recommendations used by health care providers worldwide. These recommendations are known as the NCCN Clinical Practice Guidelines in Oncology (NCCN Guidelines®).

The NCCN Guidelines for Patients plainly explain these expert recommendations, so you can talk with your care team about the best care for you.

These NCCN Guidelines for Patients are based on the NCCN Guidelines® for Hematopoietic Cell Transplantation, Version 3.2025 – September 24, 2025.

View the NCCN Guidelines for Patients free online: NCCN.org/patientguidelines

Find an NCCN Cancer Center near you: NCCN.org/cancercenters

Learn how the NCCN Guidelines for Patients are developed: NCCN.org/patient-guidelines-process

Connect with us

@NCCNorg @NCCNVideo NCCN @NCCNorg

AF883700

Supporters

NCCN Guidelines for Patients are supported by funding from the NCCN Foundation®

NCCN Foundation gratefully acknowledges the following corporate supporters for helping to make available these NCCN Guidelines for Patients: Incyte Corporation.

NCCN independently adapts, updates, and hosts the NCCN Guidelines for Patients. Our corporate supporters do not participate in the development of the NCCN Guidelines for Patients and are not responsible for the content and recommendations contained therein.

To make a gift, visit
NCCNFoundation.org/Donate

To learn more, visit online
NCCN.org/patientguidelines
or email
PatientGuidelines@NCCN.org

Contents

NCCN Foundation seeks to support the millions of patients and their families affected by a cancer diagnosis by funding and distributing NCCN Guidelines for Patients. NCCN Foundation is also committed to advancing cancer treatment by funding the nation's promising doctors at the center of innovation in cancer research. For more details and the full library of patient and caregiver resources, visit NCCN.org/patients.

National Comprehensive Cancer Network (NCCN) and NCCN Foundation
3025 Chemical Road, Suite 100, Plymouth Meeting, PA 19462 USA

1

About graft-versus-host disease

Graft-versus-host disease (GVHD) is a complication that may occur after a donor stem cell or bone marrow transplant. In GVHD, the donor's immune cells mistakenly attack your body. Read on to learn more.

How this guide can help you

Making decisions about cancer care is stressful. There's a lot to learn, and you don't know what the future holds.

Use this guide to get the information and support you need.

Patients, doctors, and other health care professionals trust the NCCN Guidelines for Patients. This guide uses clear, everyday language to explain current cancer care recommendations made by respected experts in the field. Their recommendations are based on the latest research and practices at leading cancer centers.

Your health is unique to you, so your cancer care should be, too. As you read this guide, you'll learn which treatments are likely to provide the best results for you. And you'll be better prepared to talk with your care team.

What is graft-versus-host disease?

Graft-versus-host disease (GVHD) is a side effect that happens in up to 8 out of 10 (80%) people who undergo a hematopoietic cell transplant (HCT), also known as a bone marrow transplant or stem cell transplant. An HCT replaces your stem cells and immune cells with a donor's cells.

Let's break down the term:

Graft: the donor cells that are transplanted into the body

Host: the body that receives the cells

In GVHD, the donor cells see your normal, healthy tissues as foreign and attack them.

This causes symptoms that range from mild to severe. Any area of the body can be affected. The skin, liver, and digestive tract are the most common areas affected. Other body areas may also be involved, such as the lungs, eyes, mouth, hair, nails, joints, muscles, kidneys, and genitals.

Symptoms include:
Skin rashes and mouth sores

- Pain or stiffness in joints
- Liver damage
- Dry, gritty eyes
- Diarrhea, nausea, vomiting, or difficulty swallowing
- Dryness or ulcers in genitals

- Cough, wheezing, and shortness of breath

Treatment tries to manage symptoms and prevent further damage to your body.

How is GVHD treated?

GVHD symptoms are treated with a combination of drugs such as steroids, chemotherapy, and immunotherapy. More information on the different types of drugs and other treatments for GVHD are described in Chapter 3.

Specific treatments for GVHD can vary based on the type. The next section describes them in detail.

What are the types of GVHD?

GVHD can occur within the first few months after HCT or much later.

The 2 types of GVHD differ by when symptoms occur:

Acute GVHD (aGVHD) – Develops within 100 days after transplant. It can also occur when medicines that suppress your immune system, like prednisone, are stopped. Acute GVHD primarily affects the skin, gastrointestinal (GI) tract, and liver.

Chronic GVHD (cGVHD) – Develops within 1 year after transplant. Chronic GVHD may involve the eyes, mouth, skin, joints, GI tract, lungs, and other organs. The symptoms may not be immediately obvious at first.

Each type of GVHD has a different effect on organs and tissues. Although acute and chronic GVHD usually occur at different times after transplant, it's possible to have both at the same time.

What is a hematopoietic cell transplant?

A hematopoietic cell transplant (HCT) is an intense treatment for cancer. An HCT destroys cancer cells in the bone marrow and replaces them with new, healthy blood-forming cells.

Blood stem cells

Bone marrow contains stem cells. A blood stem cell is an immature cell that can develop into a red blood cell, a white blood cell, or a platelet.

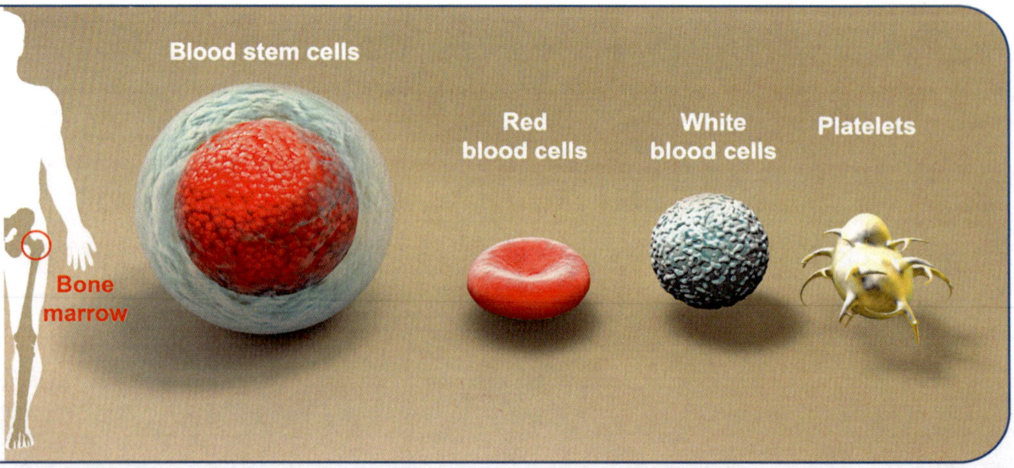

These healthy stem cells form new marrow and blood cells.

Bone marrow is the sponge-like tissue in the center of most bones. Inside your bone marrow are early blood-forming cells called blood stem cells or hematopoietic stem cells.

All types of blood cells start as blood stem cells. Once blood cells mature, they are released in your bloodstream. Normal stem cells grow and divide to make new red blood cells, white blood cells, and platelets. These cells then leave your bone marrow to perform their various jobs. These include:

- Transporting oxygen – red blood cells
- Fighting germs – white blood cells
- Stopping bleeding – platelets

An HCT may also be called a stem cell transplant or a bone marrow transplant. It occurs in 3 stages over several weeks or months:

- **Conditioning** – Before HCT, you'll receive a procedure called conditioning. Conditioning uses chemotherapy and/or radiation therapy to destroy bone marrow cells. This procedure creates room for the healthy stem cells and weakens the immune system to prevent your body from rejecting the transplanted cells.
- **Infusion** – After conditioning, you'll receive healthy stem cells through an infusion. It is a slow injection of blood products into a vein. This can take a few hours to several hours. The transplanted stem cells will travel to your bone marrow and start growing.
- **Engraftment** – New, healthy blood cells will form. This is called engraftment. It usually occurs about 2 to 4 weeks after the transplant.

Until the new, healthy blood cells form, you'll have little or no immune defense. You may need to stay in a very clean room at the hospital or be given antibiotics to prevent or treat infection.

You may receive medicine to suppress the germ-fighting portion of your body (the immune system) to prevent GVHD. While waiting for the cells to engraft, you'll likely feel tired and weak.

How can I get the best care?

Advocate for yourself. You have an important role to play in your care. Many people feel more satisfied when they actively take part in planning their cancer care.

The NCCN Guidelines for Patients will help you play a larger role in your care. Discuss the recommendations in this guide with your care team. Ask questions about your options and share your goals and concerns.

Don't know what to ask? You're not alone. That's why we include suggested questions to ask at the end of chapters.

Keep reading to find the best care for you.

2
Testing for GVHD

In order to diagnose and treat graft-versus-host disease (GVHD), you'll undergo some tests depending on your symptoms. This chapter presents an overview of the tests you might receive and what to expect.

This chapter explains the possible tests for graft-versus-host disease (GVHD). There's a good chance you won't have all of these tests, but they're listed below for your information.

If your doctor suspects you have GVHD based on your symptoms, you'll need several tests to confirm the diagnosis and exclude other possibilities before you can begin treatment. Tests are used to plan treatment and also to find out how well treatment is working.

Diagnosing GVHD

GVHD may be diagnosed based on a physical exam, blood tests, a skin exam, a biopsy, a stool sample, and possible imaging studies. Your diagnosis will determine your treatment plan.

General health tests

Physical exam

A physical exam of your body includes checking vital signs such as heart rate and blood pressure. Your provider will also look over your body and gently press on areas, feeling for your organs and lymph nodes. They may also perform a skin exam.

Medical history

A medical history is a record of all health issues and treatments you've had in your life. Be prepared to list any illness or injury, and when it happened.

Bring a list of old and new medicines and any over-the-counter medicines, herbal remedies, or supplements you take. Tell your health care provider about any symptoms you have.

Guide 1 Testing for GVHD
Medical history and physical exam
Complete blood count (CBC)
Metabolic panel
Liver function tests
Hepatitis panel
Skin exam
Fecal analysis
Biopsy
Imaging (CT, MRI, ultrasound)

All of this information is needed to find out your current state of health and whether you have symptoms. This information helps your care team figure out which tests you may need first. Another goal of the medical history is to uncover clues about any potential treatment that could cause you harm.

Blood tests

Blood tests check for signs of disease and how well your organs are working. They require a sample of your blood, which is removed through a needle placed into your arm.

If you know your veins are difficult to find, let the lab tech know, and they can get a machine that will help find your veins. This way, you'll get fewer pokes from the needle, and it's less stressful.

Complete blood count

A complete blood count, or CBC, measures the levels of red blood cells, white blood cells, and platelets in your blood. Low blood counts don't necessarily mean you have acute GVHD (aGVHD). But it's common for patients with GVHD to develop low blood counts.

Metabolic panel

Kidney function and electrolytes can be affected by side effects from medicine or if you're dehydrated from having diarrhea GVHD can also impair kidney function. A basic metabolic panel checks kidney function and electrolytes in the blood.

Liver function tests

Liver function tests measure chemicals made or processed by the liver. Levels that are too high or too low signal that the liver is not working well and can be a sign of GVHD.

One chemical measured is bilirubin. If the liver isn't working as it should, there may be too much bilirubin in the blood. Too much bilirubin causes jaundice, a yellowing of the eyes and skin. It might also cause itchy skin and dark-colored urine.

Hepatitis panel

Hepatitis is the inflammation of the liver. Sometimes this inflammation is caused by viruses, such as hepatitis A, hepatitis B, and hepatitis C. Hepatitis causes the liver to not work as it should.

A hepatitis panel can tell your treatment team if you've had hepatitis in the past or if you have it today. Certain treatments used for GVHD, such as immunosuppressive therapies, can reactivate hepatitis B in the blood.

Skin exam

Skin conditions such as rashes, lesions, bumps, and dry or peeling skin are common in GVHD. Find an experienced health care provider, such as a dermatologist, to conduct a thorough skin exam. Expect a head-to-toe examination.

A skin lesion is a change in color or texture. Keeping a photo journal might help track your skin changes.

Skin lesions include erythroderma, papules, papulonodules, patches, plaques, and ulcers.

Erythroderma

Erythroderma can look like redness or sunburn on people with lighter-colored skin and blotches of various colors on people with darker-colored skin.

Papule

A papule is a very small, solid lump that might look like a very small pimple. Papules are usually found in groups. They may be red, purple, brown, or pink.

Papulonodule

A papulonodule is a combination of papules and nodules found on the skin. Nodules are more raised than papules.

Patch

A patch is a flat, thin, pink or red lesion of any size that forms on the skin. Patches may be dry, scaly, or itchy and may look like eczema or psoriasis. They can be lighter in color than surrounding skin or brown in people with darker skin. Patches may sometimes become plaques (hard, raised lesions) on the skin.

Plaque

A plaque is a raised or hardened lesion of any size that forms on the skin. Plaques may be red, scaly, or itchy and may look like eczema or psoriasis. They can appear on up to half (50%) of the body in serious cases.

Skin lesions

A papule is a very small, solid bump. A plaque is a raised or hardened lesion that forms on the skin, larger than a papule.

Credit: Madhero88, CC BY-SA 3.0, via Wikimedia Commons

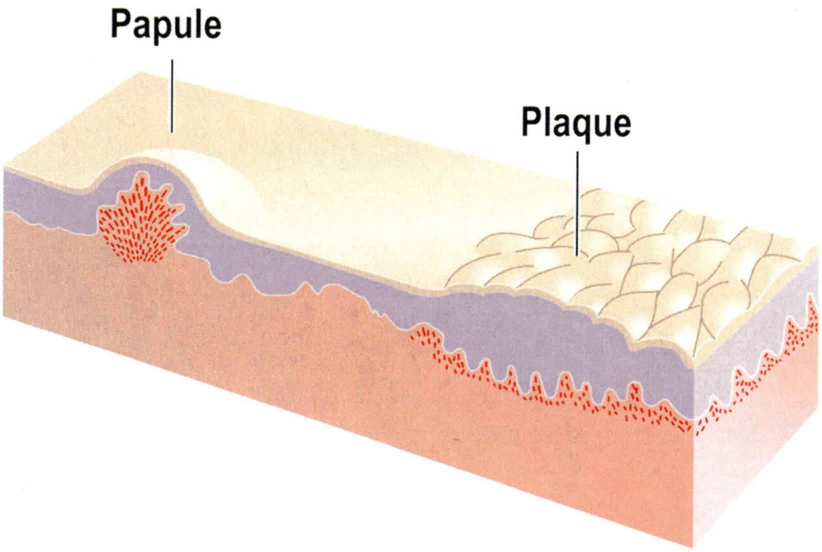

Ulcer

A skin ulcer is an open sore or wound on the skin caused by poor blood flow. Ulcers caused by GVHD can also be found in the mouth or on the genitals.

Fecal analysis

Feces (poop) is made up of undigested food, bacteria, mucus, and cells from the lining of the intestines. Since GVHD might affect the digestive tract, symptoms such as diarrhea or abdominal pain are important to watch.

Infection in the bowels can also cause these symptoms. So if you're having diarrhea and GVHD is suspected, your care providers will also test for gastrointestinal (GI) infections.

For this test, you'll provide a sample of your poop. You'll be given a special container with a lid to take home and gloves for handling the container. Speak with your health care provider about how you should collect the fecal sample and any special instructions.

Biopsy

A biopsy is the removal of a sample of tissue or a group of cells for testing. It's an important part of an accurate diagnosis.

After the procedure, your sample should be reviewed by a pathologist who is an expert in

Erythroderma

Erythroderma is severe inflammation of most of the body's skin surface. It can look like sunburn or large splotches.

Credit: James Heilman, MD, CC BY-SA 4.0, via Wikimedia Commons

Credit: Mohammad2018, CC BY-SA 4.0, via Wikimedia Commons

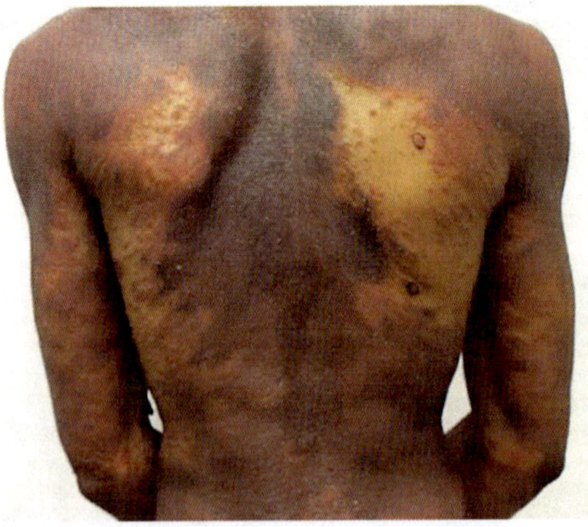

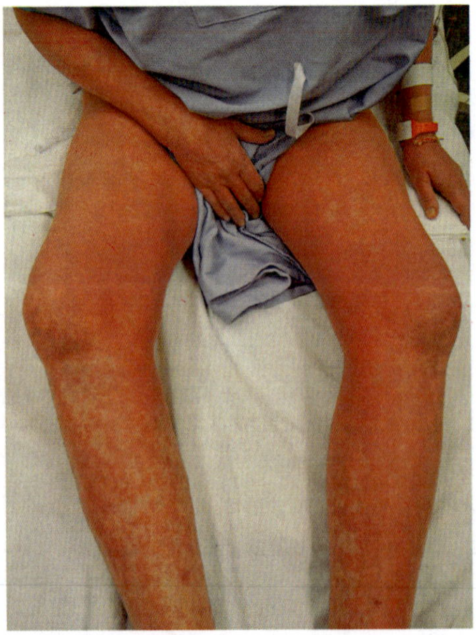

the diagnosis of GVHD. This review is often referred to as a histology, histopathology, or hematopathology review. The pathologist will note the overall appearance and the size, shape, and type of your cells.

Biopsies of the skin, GI tract, liver, or other organs might be done to confirm GVHD.

Skin biopsy

If you have skin lesions, a sample of your lesion may be removed and tested to plan treatment. The area will be numbed with medicine before it's removed.

GI biopsy

A GI biopsy is often performed to confirm a diagnosis of gastrointestinal acute GVHD. A biopsy might be done during a procedure that looks inside your GI tract, like an endoscopy, colonoscopy, or flexible sigmoidoscopy.

In an endoscopy, a long, tube-like device equipped with a tiny video camera is guided down the throat into the esophagus, stomach, and upper parts of the small intestine. The endoscope is used to inspect the lining of these organs. It also checks for any signs of cancer or other abnormalities, such as dilated blood vessels or ulcers. This can also be referred to as an upper GI endoscopy or duodenoscopy.

In a colonoscopy and flexible sigmoidoscopy, a device is inserted into your rear end (rectum) to inspect inside the colon.

For any of these biopsy tests, you'll be under general anesthesia (in a sleep-like state) for the procedure.

Liver biopsy

In a liver biopsy, a needle may be inserted through the skin of your abdomen to remove a liver sample. Or it may be inserted through a large vein in your neck, called the jugular vein, and threaded down to a vein near your liver.

You won't feel any pain during this procedure. You'll be given medicine to help numb you and put you to sleep if needed.

Imaging

Imaging tests take pictures of the inside of your body to look for illness, injury, or other conditions. A radiologist, an expert in interpreting test images, will write a report and send it to your health care provider. Your test results will be discussed with you.

X-ray

An x-ray uses low-dose radiation to take pictures of the inside of your body. A chest x-ray is used to check for infection in your lungs.

CT scan

A CT or CAT scan uses x-rays and computer technology to take pictures of the inside of your body, such as in your stomach/ intestines or your liver, which can have GVHD symptoms.

MRI scan

An MRI scan uses radio waves and powerful magnets to take pictures of the inside of your body. MRI scans tend to be of higher quality and may be used in place of CT scans.

MRIs don't use x-rays or radiation, so they can be taken more frequently.

Ultrasound

An ultrasound uses high-energy sound waves to form pictures of the inside of your body. This is similar to the sonogram used for pregnancy. Sometimes an ultrasound is used to guide a biopsy of your liver or anything else that's under your skin. For this procedure, a probe will be pressed onto your abdomen.

An ultrasound is painless and doesn't use x-rays or radiation, so it can be repeated as often as needed.

Performance status

Performance status is an evaluation of a person's general level of fitness and ability to perform daily tasks. Your care team uses this evaluation to get a sense of the level of treatment you may be able to handle and whether you may be eligible for a clinical trial. In general, a person with a higher performance status can tolerate more intensive treatment.

"You don't have control over the past or future, but you do have control over this moment now. Live for the moment each and every day."

Key points

- Accurate testing is needed to diagnose and treat graft-versus-host disease (GVHD).
- Blood tests check for signs of disease and how well organs are working.
- Skin conditions such as rashes, lesions, and dry or peeling skin are common in GVHD.
- A biopsy is the removal of a sample of tissue or group of cells for testing. It may be an important part of diagnosing GVHD.
- Depending on your symptoms, a biopsy of your skin, liver, gastrointestinal (GI) tract, or other organs may be necessary.
- Imaging tests take pictures of the inside of your body to look for signs of GVHD.
- Performance status is a person's general level of fitness and ability to perform daily tasks.

Questions to ask

- Is there a cancer center or hospital nearby that specializes in GVHD?
- What tests are needed? What other tests do you recommend?
- What will you do to make me comfortable during testing?

What's next?

Once GVHD is appropriately diagnosed, you'll receive treatment. The types of treatment available are discussed in the next chapter.

3
Types of treatment

Once graft-versus-host disease (GVHD) is confirmed, you'll receive recommendations for treatment. Together, you and your health care provider will choose a treatment plan that is best for you. This chapter describes treatments commonly recommended for GVHD.

A normal treatment plan for GVHD uses medication to suppress the immune system. This prevents your immune system from attacking the donor cells.

Immunosuppressants

Immunosuppressive therapy is a type of drug therapy that lowers the body's immune response. This helps to prevent the donor immune cells from attacking your healthy tissues. It uses materials made either by the body or in a laboratory to improve, target, or restore immune system function.

Immunosuppressants can be topical (applied to body surface, with local effect) or systemic (taken as pill, IV, etc. and affects whole body).

Some immunosuppressants used to treat graft-versus-host disease (GVHD) include:

- Steroids
- Calcineurin inhibitors (such as cyclosporine and tacrolimus)
- Mycophenolate mofetil

Steroids

Corticosteroids, or steroids, are lab-made immunosuppressants used to reduce inflammation in many conditions. In GVHD, they're used to stop activated donor immune cells from harming your body.

Steroids can be placed on the skin as an ointment or gel, inhaled through the mouth, used as a mouth rinse, taken as a pill, or given as an infusion through an IV needle placed in your arm. They each work differently to treat the side effects of GVHD.

Steroids can cause short-term and long-term side effects. Ask your care team about possible side effects.

Usually, steroids are used as a first-line treatment for both acute and chronic GVHD.

Calcineurin inhibitors

A calcineurin inhibitor is used for the prevention and treatment of GVHD. Types include cyclosporine, tacrolimus ointment (Protopic), tacrolimus (Prograf), and pimecrolimus (topical only). They can be used as a pill, intravenously (IV), as an ointment, or as an oral rinse.

Mycophenolate mofetil

Mycophenolate mofetil (CellCept) is an immunosuppressive agent used to prevent organ rejection in people with organ transplants. If you've received or likely will receive a bone marrow transplant, then you'll probably receive this medicine.

Immunotherapy

When a medicine is made to trigger the body's defense system, we call this immunotherapy. The most common immunotherapy used in GVHD is extracorporeal photopheresis.

Extracorporeal photopheresis

Extracorporeal photopheresis is a type of immunotherapy used to treat GVHD. In this procedure, blood is circulated outside the body through a filter that separates the white blood cells from the rest of the blood.

Then, the white blood cells are combined with a light-sensitive agent and exposed to ultraviolet (UV) light to activate the medicine, which kills the immune cells. Lastly, the treated cells are reinfused back into your body.

Interleukin-2 (IL-2)

Another immunotherapy that is used for chronic steroid-refractory GVHD is interleukin-2 (IL-2). This is a naturally occurring protein in the immune system that stimulates the growth of germ-fighting T cells.

Systemic therapy

Systemic therapy is treatment that affects the whole body. It's usually given by mouth as a pill or tablet, or through a needle inserted into a vein.

Guide 2 Steroids for GVHD
Prednisone
Methylprednisolone (Solu-Medrol)
Beclomethasone dipropionate
Budesonide (Entocort EC, Ortikos, Uceris)
Budesonide (Pulmicort Flexhaler, Pulmicort Respules)
Fluticasone (Flovent HFA, Flovent Diskus)
Hydrocortisone cream or ointment (1% or 2.5%)
Triamcinolone cream or ointment
Clobetasol ointment (Cormax, Embeline, or Temovate)
Dexamethasone

Types of systemic therapy used to treat GVHD include:

- Antibiotics
- Antihistamines
- Biologics
- Targeted therapy
- Topical steroids
- Phototherapy
- Chemotherapy

Ask your health care provider about the goal of systemic therapy and why one therapy might be chosen over another. It might be related to your symptoms, cost, toxicity, or availability. But don't forget that your preferences also matter.

Systemic therapies can fall into more than one category. The types described on the following pages provide a general overview. Not all possible drugs are listed.

Antihistamines

Antihistamines are a type of drug that blocks the action of histamines, which can cause reactions like fever, itching, sneezing, a runny nose, and watery eyes. Antihistamines can control itchy skin, watery eyes, and other symptoms of GVHD.

Biologics

A biologic is a drug made from a living organism or its products. Etanercept (Enbrel) and infliximab (Remicade) are biologics that stop or slow inflammation. Other examples of biologics used for GVHD include antithymocyte globulin (ATG), alpha-1 proteinase inhibitor (AAT), basiliximab (Simulect), tocilizumab (Actemra), rituximab (Rituxan), and vedolizumab (Entyvio).

Team approach

Treatment decisions should involve a multidisciplinary team of doctors, health care workers, and social care professionals with knowledge and experience with GVHD.

Your team might include:

- **A hematologist** is an expert in blood diseases and cancers.
- **A dermatologist** specializes in the diagnosis and treatment of skin diseases.
- **A pathologist** analyzes the cells, tissues, and organs removed during a biopsy and provides information about biomarker and genetic testing.
- **A diagnostic radiologist** reads the results of x-rays and other imaging tests.
- **An interventional radiologist** performs needle biopsies and places ports for treatment.
- **A medical oncologist** treats cancer in adults using systemic therapy.
- **A radiation oncologist** prescribes and plans radiation therapy to treat cancer.
- **An anesthesiologist** gives anesthesia, a medicine so you don't feel pain during procedures.

Biosimilars

A biosimilar might be used in place of some drugs. A biosimilar is a drug that is very much like one that has been approved by the U.S. Food and Drug Administration (FDA). It must be used in the same way and at the same dose as the other drug.

Targeted therapy

Targeted therapy focuses on specific or unique features of cells throughout the body. Ibrutinib (Imbruvica), ruxolitinib (Jakafi), belumosudil (Rezurock), alemtuzumab (Campath or Lemtrada), abatacept (Orencia), axatilimab-csfr (Niktimvo), and imatinib (Gleevec) are targeted therapies.

mTOR inhibitors such as sirolimus (Rapamune) are also targeted therapies.

Ruxolitinib is used in both acute and chronic GVHD that did not have a good response to steroids. Ibrutinib and belumosudil are used in both acute and chronic GVHD.

Skin-directed therapy

Types of therapy focused on the skin include topical steroids and phototherapy.

Topical steroids

Topical steroids are put on the surface of the skin and are used to treat skin conditions due to GVHD. These include lotions, creams, gels, and ointments.

Topical steroids used to treat GVHD include:

- Clobetasol propionate
- Hydrocortisone
- Triamcinolone acetonide (Triderm)
- Tacrolimus ointment (Protopic)

Phototherapy

Phototherapy uses UV light to treat skin lesions in GVHD. This treatment might be given to treat severe skin-only GVHD. Photochemotherapy combines psoralen with ultraviolet light A (UVA).

Psoralen is a type of medicine taken as a pill that causes your skin to be sensitive to light. After taking psoralen, the skin is exposed to long-wave UVA light, which reduces inflammation and slows skin cell production.

UV can increase your risk of some skin cancers. So phototherapy may not be a good choice for those with a history of squamoproliferative skin neoplasms, basal cell carcinomas, or melanoma.

For more information, see *NCCN Guidelines for Patients: Basal Cell Skin Cancer* or *NCCN Guidelines for Patients: Melanoma*, available at NCCN.org/patientguidelines and on the NCCN Patient Guides for Cancer app.

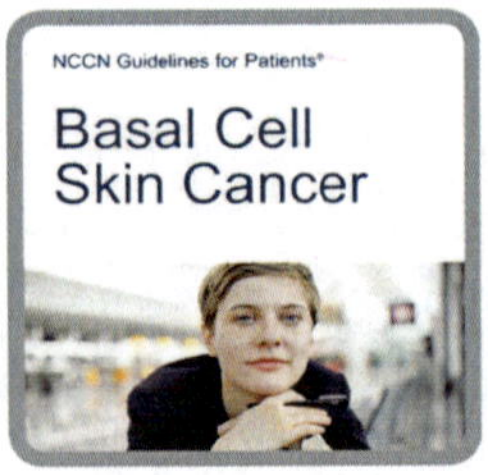

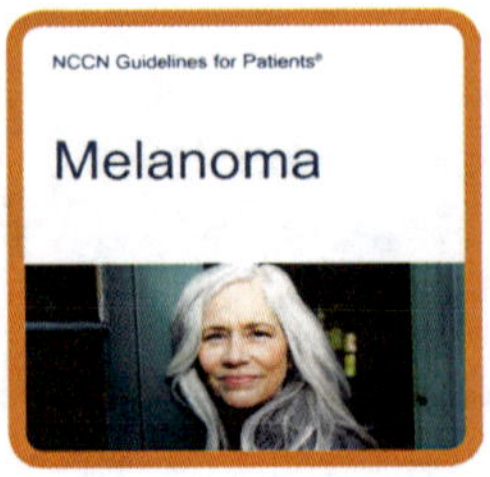

Chemotherapy

Chemotherapy kills fast-growing cells throughout the body, including cancer cells and normal cells.

Methotrexate (Otrexup) is used to prevent GVHD following a hematopoietic cell transplant (HCT). This medicine stops the cells from dividing and making new cells. Since methotrexate may cause mouth sores, good oral care is very important.

Melphalan (Alkeran), cyclophosphamide (Cytoxan), and pentostatin (Nipent) are other chemotherapies that may be used for GVHD prevention.

Supportive care

Supportive care is an important part of cancer care. The goal is to improve your quality of life during and after cancer treatment. Supportive care is for everyone with cancer and their families, not just for those at the end of life. It's also known as palliative care.

Supportive care includes a wide range of services. Supportive care prevents or manages the symptoms of cancer and the side effects of cancer treatment, like pain and cancer-related fatigue. It also addresses the mental, social, emotional, and spiritual concerns faced by people with cancer.

Supportive care provides help with additional needs, such as:

- Making treatment decisions
- Coordinating your care
- Paying for care
- Planning for advance care and end of life

Read more about the types of support you may receive in *NCCN Guidelines for Patients: Palliative Care*, available at NCCN.org/patientguidelines and on the NCCN Patient Guides for Cancer app.

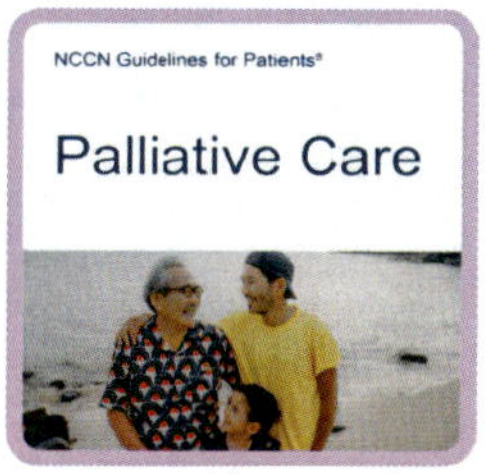

Before your HCT, you likely had many rounds of systemic therapy, and possibly radiation therapy, to treat your cancer. This weakens your body.

An HCT further weakens your body. You may also have other serious health issues like high blood pressure or diabetes that may complicate recovery.

Take care of yourself by eating well, drinking plenty of fluids, exercising, and doing things that make you feel energized. Strength is needed to sustain you while being treated for GVHD.

Supportive care is also for treating symptoms of GVHD, including diarrhea, distress, fatigue, nausea and vomiting, appetite problems, and pain.

Antibiotics

Infections occur more frequently and are more severe in people with a weakened immune system. An HCT weakens the body's natural defense against infections.

If not treated early, infections can be fatal. Infections can be caused by viruses, fungi, or bacteria. Antibiotics can treat bacterial infections. Antifungal medicines can treat fungal infections. You may be given antiviral drugs to prevent viral infections.

Azithromycin (Zithromax, also known as a Z-Pak) is an antibiotic that might be used to treat lung issues in chronic GVHD.

Diarrhea

Diarrhea is frequent and watery poops or bowel movements. Your care team will tell you how to manage diarrhea and may recommend prescription medicines to help stop it. Drink lots of fluids. Changes to your diet might help.

Over-the-counter diarrhea medicines include loperamide (Imodium) or bismuth subsalicylate (Kaopectate or Pepto-Bismol), but consult with your care team if these aren't helping you.

Talk to your care team if you see anything unusual in your poop, such as blood.

Distress

Distress is an unpleasant experience of a mental, physical, social, or spiritual nature. It can affect how you feel, think, and act. This might include feelings of sadness, fear, helplessness, worry, anger, and guilt.

Depression, anxiety, and sleeping problems are common in those with GVHD and people with cancer in general. Talk to your health care provider and the people in your life about how you are feeling.

There are services and people who can help you. Support and counseling services are available. You can find support groups online at www.cancercare.org/support_groups. You can also ask your care team for an oncology social worker.

Remember, you're not alone.

For more information, see *NCCN Guidelines for Patients: Distress During Cancer Care*, available at NCCN.org/patientguidelines. and on the NCCN Patient Guides for Cancer app.

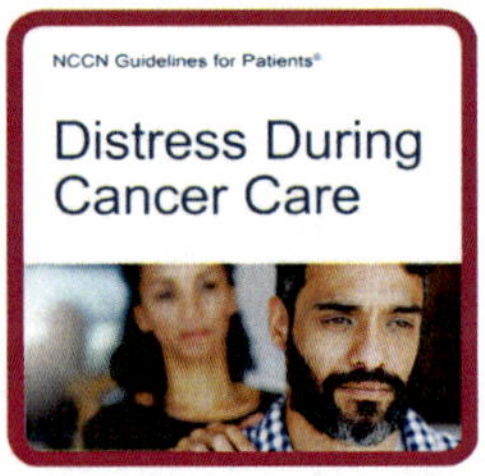

Fatigue

Fatigue is being extremely tired and unable to function due to a lack of energy. Fatigue may be a sign of GVHD. There are treatments for fatigue.

Let your care team know how you are feeling and if fatigue is getting in the way of doing the things you enjoy. Eating a balanced diet, exercising, yoga, and massage therapy can help. You might be referred to a nutritionist or dietitian to help with fatigue.

Nausea and vomiting

Nausea and vomiting might be a sign of GVHD. You'll be given medicine to treat nausea and vomiting. Ondansetron (Zofran) is an example of a medicine that can help people with nausea and vomiting.

Trouble eating

Sometimes, side effects from GVHD might cause you to feel not hungry or sick to your stomach (nauseated). You might have a sore mouth.

Healthy eating is important during treatment. It includes eating a balanced diet, eating the right amount of food, and drinking enough fluids. A registered dietitian who is an expert in nutrition and food can help. Speak to your care team if you have trouble eating or maintaining your weight.

Pain

Pain is common in GVHD. It might be caused by nausea and vomiting or abdominal cramps from diarrhea. Pain can also occur in the eyes, the joints and muscles, or the mouth. Tell your care team about any pain or discomfort you have. You might meet with a palliative care specialist or pain specialist to manage your pain.

Clinical trials

A clinical trial is a type of medical research study. After being developed and tested in a lab, potential new ways of fighting cancer need to be studied in people.

If found to be safe and effective in a clinical trial, a drug, device, or treatment approach may be approved by the U.S. Food and Drug Administration (FDA).

Everyone with cancer should carefully consider all of the treatment options available for their cancer type, including standard treatments and clinical trials. Talk to your doctor about whether a clinical trial may make sense for you.

Phases

Most cancer clinical trials focus on treatment and are done in phases.

- **Phase 1** trials study the safety and side effects of an investigational drug or treatment approach.
- **Phase 2** trials study how well the drug or approach works against a specific type of cancer.
- **Phase 3** trials test the drug or approach against a standard treatment. If the results are good, it may be approved by the FDA.
- **Phase 4** trials study the safety and benefit of an FDA-approved treatment.

Finding a clinical trial

In the United States

NCCN Cancer Centers
NCCN.org/cancercenters

The National Cancer Institute (NCI)
cancer.gov/about-cancer/treatment/clinical-trials/search

Worldwide

The U.S. National Library of Medicine (NLM)
clinicaltrials.gov

Need help finding a clinical trial?

NCI's Cancer Information Service (CIS)
1.800.4.CANCER (1.800.422.6237)
cancer.gov/contact

Who can enroll?

It depends on the clinical trial's rules, called eligibility criteria. The rules may be about age, cancer type and stage, treatment history, or general health. They ensure that participants are alike in specific ways and that the trial is as safe as possible for the participants.

Informed consent

Clinical trials are managed by a research team. This group of experts will review the study with you in detail, including its purpose and the risks and benefits of joining. All of this information is also provided in an informed consent form. Read the form carefully and ask questions before signing it. Take time to discuss it with people you trust. Keep in mind that you can leave and seek treatment outside of the clinical trial at any time.

Will I get a placebo?

Placebos (inactive versions of real medicines) are almost never used alone in cancer clinical trials. It is common to receive either a placebo with a standard treatment, or a new drug with a standard treatment. You will be informed, verbally and in writing, if a placebo is part of a clinical trial before you enroll.

Are clinical trials free?

There is no fee to enroll in a clinical trial. The study sponsor pays for research-related costs, including the study drug. But you may need to pay for other services, like transportation or childcare, due to extra appointments. During the trial, you will continue to receive standard cancer care. This care is often covered by insurance.

Urinary-derived human chorionic gonadotropin/epidermal growth factor

A medicine being tested in clinical trials for the treatment of GVHD is urinary-derived human chorionic gonadotropin/epidermal growth factor (uhCG/EGF), which is showing promising results as of this writing. You may receive this medication if it's available in your area and you need it (see more information in the next chapter).

Many other clinical trials in the field of GVHD seek to make dosing existing medicines easier and to test new medicines.

Key points

- Treatment decisions should involve a multidisciplinary team of health care providers from different professional backgrounds who have expertise and experience with GVHD.
- Steroids are usually the first-line therapy for GVHD.
- Skin-directed therapy includes topical therapy and phototherapy.
- Systemic therapy is a treatment that affects the whole body. It's usually given by mouth or through a needle inserted into a vein (intravenously or IV).
- Chemotherapy kills fast-growing cells throughout the body, including cancer cells and normal cells.
- Immunosuppressants are drugs or biologic products used to prevent or stop the donor's immune system from harming your body.
- Supportive care is health care that relieves symptoms caused by GVHD and improves quality of life.

Questions to ask

- What are my treatment options?
- Will my age, health, and other factors affect my options?
- Am I a candidate for a clinical trial?
- What are the side effects of systemic therapy? Topical therapy? Steroids?
- How long will these side effects last? Do any side effects lessen or worsen in severity over time?

What's next?

The treatments you may receive are determined based on the type of GVHD that you're experiencing. The first of the two types, acute GVHD (aGVHD), is discussed in the next chapter.

4 Acute GVHD

Acute graft-versus-host disease (aGVHD) is a complication from a donor stem cell transplant. Treatment aims to suppress the immune response and manage symptoms.

In acute graft-versus-host disease (GVHD/aGVHD), the cells you received from the hematopoietic cell transplant (HCT) attack areas of your body such as the skin, liver, and gastrointestinal (GI) tract. You might have a skin rash, diarrhea, nausea, vomiting, and liver function issues. There may be more than one of these symptoms in more severe cases.

Tests will be done to rule out non-GVHD causes. Biopsies of the skin, GI tract, liver, or other organs might be done to confirm GVHD.

Staging

After diagnosis, your GVHD will be given a stage. This stage notes how severe the GVHD is. It will be used to make treatment decisions.

In acute GVHD, each organ receives a stage that is factored together to assign a grade to the disease. This section describes the staging process.

The skin is given a stage based on the amount of body surface area involved.

The GI tract is given a stage based on the amount of diarrhea or number of poops or bowel movements per day.

The liver is given an individual organ stage based on the rise in your bilirubin level.

Stage 1

Stage 1 aGVHD means you have one of the following:

- Rash on less than 25% (or one-quarter) of your skin
- Bilirubin levels between 2 and 3 mg/dL
- Persistent nausea or greater than 500 mL of diarrhea

Treatment

Treatments for stage 1 aGVHD include continuing or restarting an immunosuppressive agent with topical steroids, or observation. Your care team may simply observe you if no symptoms are found or your rash is stable (unchanged).

Response

If your stage 1 aGVHD improves with treatment, your dose of the immunosuppressive agent will be reduced until you're not taking it anymore.

No response

If aGVHD doesn't improve with treatment, your health care provider may refer you to a clinical trial or recommend you to continue with topical steroids.

Progression

If the medicine doesn't seem to help or it makes your condition worse, you may develop higher stages of GVHD or require more intensive treatments.

Stages 2, 3, and 4

In stage 2 aGVHD, you have one or more of the following:

- Rash on up to half of your skin
- Bilirubin levels between 3 and 6 mg/dL
- Diarrhea greater than 1000 mL/day

In stage 3 aGVHD, you have one or more of the following:

- Rash on over half of your skin
- Bilirubin levels between 6 and 15 mg/dL
- Diarrhea greater than 1500 mL/day

In stage 4 aGVHD, you have one or more of the following:

- Erythroderma with blisters
- Bilirubin levels greater than 15 mg/dL
- Severe abdominal pain and diarrhea or constipation

Treatment

Treatment for aGVHD stages 2 through 4 may include:

- Continue or restart the original immunosuppressive agent. Your dose may be increased from what you were originally taking or are currently taking.
- Clinical trial
- Systemic steroids with or without topical steroids
- Sirolimus, also known as rapamycin (Rapamune)

Depending on your symptoms, you may be given steroid pills or creams to use at home, or you may be admitted to the hospital for intravenous (IV) treatments.

Response

If your symptoms improve, then you'll be tapered off steroids until you're no longer taking them. Since long-term steroid use causes health issues and risk for infection, you'll be tapered off steroids as soon as possible.

Some people may remain on low-dose steroids to maintain a healthy response. Side effects will be managed by your care team as they come up.

No response

If your symptoms don't improve, your health care provider might:

- Refer you for a clinical trial
- Add a systemic agent to steroids

If aGVHD doesn't respond to treatment, then you'll be treated for steroid-refractory disease.

Refractory means resistant to treatment. In steroid-refractory disease, GVHD stops responding to or worsens during standard steroid treatment. Steroid-refractory disease happens in about half of people with acute GVHD. Steroid-refractory acute GVHD (SR-aGVHD) is very serious and can be life-threatening.

Participation in a clinical trial is encouraged if available. Or SR-aGVHD can be treated with a steroid and additional systemic therapy, which may be given as a pill or IV. Often, your original immunosuppressant will be combined with the systemic therapy found in **Guide 3**.

Guide 3 Steroid-refractory acute GVHD systemic therapy
Ruxolitinib (preferred)
Alemtuzumab
Alpha-1 antitrypsin (AAT)
Anti-thymocyte globulin (ATG)
Basiliximab
Calcineurin inhibitors
Etanercept
Extracorporeal photopheresis (ECP) (PUVA [psoralen and ultraviolet A] may be an option in some cases)
Infliximab
mTOR inhibitors (eg, sirolimus)
Mycophenolate mofetil
Pentostatin
Tocilizumab
Urinary-derived human chorionic gonadotropin/epidermal growth factor (uhCG/EGF)
Vedolizumab

Key points

- Acute graft-versus-host disease (aGVHD) is a complication from a donor stem cell transplant. It typically develops soon after a transplant.
- In aGVHD, the donor cells attack areas of your body such as the skin, liver, and gastrointestinal (GI) tract. You might have a skin rash, diarrhea, nausea, vomiting, and liver function issues.
- In aGVHD, each organ is staged individually.
- Treatment options for stage 1 aGVHD may include an immunosuppressive agent and/or topical steroids or observation.
- Treatment options for aGVHD stages 2 through 4 may include immunosuppressive agents, a clinical trial, systemic steroids with or without topical steroids, or sirolimus.
- In steroid-refractory disease, GVHD stops responding to or worsens on steroid treatment. Steroid-refractory acute GVHD (SR-aGVHD) is treated with a steroid and additional systemic therapy.
- Depending on the severity (how bad) of your symptoms, you may be treated at home with pills and topical creams, or you may need to be admitted to the hospital for intravenous (IV) treatments.

Questions to ask

- What stage of acute GVHD do I have?
- Should I inspect my skin regularly? If so, how often?
- If I notice any changes in my skin, who should I call? When?
- Will keeping a diary and photo journal help? What should I include in my diary? How often should I take photos?

What's next?

Acute GVHD can go away with treatment, and another form of GVHD can emerge more than a year later.

People who don't develop acute GVHD may still develop GVHD within a year afterward. This is called chronic GVHD (cGVHD) and is discussed in the next chapter.

5

Chronic GVHD

Chronic graft-versus-host disease (cGVHD) is a complication from a donor stem cell transplant. It typically develops within 1 year of the transplant and will require long-term monitoring. Treatment aims to control symptoms, avoid organ damage, and improve quality of life.

Before starting treatment, a diagnosis of chronic graft-versus host disease (cGVHD) will be confirmed, and a disease grade will be given. While a biopsy may be done to confirm chronic GVHD, a biopsy is not always possible or necessary.

Chronic GVHD can affect the following areas of the body:

- Eyes
- Mouth and esophagus
- Lungs
- Liver
- Genitals and urinary system
- Kidneys
- Joints, skin, and muscles

Oral health care

Chronic GVHD can cause problems in your mouth. Symptoms often include sensitivity and pain, dry mouth, changes in taste, and difficulty opening your mouth. Seek care by a dental professional if symptoms persist or worsen.

There are steps you can take to prevent symptoms, including:

- Having dental check-ups every 6 months
- Brushing your teeth, gums, and tongue after meals and before bed
- Using a toothpaste with fluoride and an alcohol-free mouthwash
- Flossing your teeth gently every day
- Using mouth rinses (baking soda and salt in warm water, followed by plain water rinse)
- Cleaning, brushing, and rinsing dentures after meals
- Making sure dentures fit well

What's a grade?

A grade is a rating or score given to specific signs or symptoms of GVHD (see *Chapter 1: About graft-versus-host disease* for a list of symptoms of GVHD).

Grading is based on your performance status and the area(s) of the body that have been affected. A score of zero (0) means there are no symptoms or signs. Severe symptoms or signs are given the highest score of 3.

Treatment

Treatment for chronic GVHD aims to control symptoms, avoid organ damage, and improve quality of life.

Treatment is based on symptoms. Options may include one or more of the following:

- Clinical trial
- Continue or restart the original immunosuppressive therapy
- Systemic corticosteroids (methylprednisolone or prednisone) or sirolimus (Rapamune) with prednisone
- Topical steroids as needed (such as triamcinolone or clobetasol), topical estrogen for vulvovaginal GVHD, topical tacrolimus, or dexamethasone mouth rinse for oral GVHD
- Inhaled steroid (examples include budesonide or fluticasone)
- Azithromycin (Zithromax) for lung involvement (those with progression or worsening of lung cGVHD following 2 to 3 lines of therapy may be evaluated for lung transplant)
- Montelukast (Singulair) for if your breathing is affected

Since long-term steroid use causes health issues and risk for infection, you'll be tapered off steroids when possible. Some people may remain on low-dose steroids for as long as possible.

If cGVHD doesn't respond to treatment, then you'll be treated for steroid-refractory disease.

Steroid-refractory cGVHD

Refractory means resistant to treatment. Steroid-refractory disease happens in about half of people with chronic GVHD. Steroid-refractory chronic GVHD (SR-cGVHD) is very serious and can be life-threatening. Participation in a clinical trial is encouraged, if available.

In SR-cGVHD, GVHD stops responding to or worsens on steroid treatment. To get your disease under control, another systemic therapy is added to the steroid treatment. Often, your original immunosuppressant is combined with a systemic therapy found in **Guide 4**.

Guide 4 Steroid-refractory chronic GVHD systemic therapy
Ruxolitinib (preferred)
Abatacept
Alemtuzumab
Axatilimab-csfr
Belumosudil
Calcineurin inhibitors
Etanercept
Extracorporeal photopheresis (ECP) (PUVA [psoralen and ultraviolet A] may be an option in some cases)
Hydroxychloroquine
Ibrutinib
Imatinib
Interleukin-2 (IL-2)
Low-Dose Methotrexate
mTOR inhibitors (eg, sirolimus)
Mycophenolate mofetil
Pentostatin
Rituximab or its biosimilar

Key points

- Before starting treatment, a diagnosis of chronic graft-versus-host disease (cGVHD) will be confirmed and a disease grade will be given.
- When possible, a biopsy will be done to confirm chronic GVHD (cGVHD).
- Grading is a rating or score given to the amount of signs of symptoms of GVHD.
- Treatment for chronic GVHD aims to control symptoms, avoid organ damage, and improve quality of life.
- In steroid-refractory chronic GVHD (SR-cGVHD), GVHD stops responding to or worsens on steroid treatment. More systemic therapy will be added to your treatment.
- Anyone with cGVHD is encouraged to participate in a clinical trial.

We want your feedback!

Our goal is to provide helpful and easy-to-understand information on cancer. Take our survey to let us know what we got right and what we could do better.
NCCN.org/patients/feedback

Questions to ask

- What is the outlook for chronic GVHD?
- Are there any clinical trials for patients with chronic GVHD like me?
- Is the chronic GVHD steroid-refractory? If so, how do we proceed?

6
Other resources

Want to learn more? Here's how you can get additional help.

What else to know

This book can help you improve your cancer care. It plainly explains expert recommendations and suggests questions to ask your care team. But it's not the only resource that you have.

You're welcome to receive as much information and help as you need. Many people are interested in learning more about:

- Details on how treatments work
- Symptoms of graft-versus-host disease (GVHD) or side effects of medicines
- Getting financial help
- Finding a care provider who is an expert in GVHD
- Coping with symptoms and side effects of GVHD treatment

What else to do

Your health care center can help you with next steps. They often have on-site resources to help meet your needs and find answers to your questions. Health care centers can also inform you of resources in your community.

In addition to help from your providers, the resources listed in the next section provide support for many people like yourself. Look through the list and visit the provided websites to learn more about these organizations.

Where to get help

Blood & Marrow Transplant Information Network (BMT InfoNet)
BMTInfoNet.org

Blood Cancer United
Bloodcancerunited.org

CancerCare
Cancercare.org

Imerman Angels
Imermanangels.org

National Bone Marrow Transplant Link (nbmtLINK)
nbmtlink.org

PAN Foundation
Panfoundation.org

Triage Cancer
Triagecancer.org

Questions to ask

- Are there support groups for people with GVHD?
- How can I get involved in GVHD research and philanthropy?
- What can I do to help others with GVHD?

Words to know

acute
A sudden, severe, short-term illness.

biopsy
Removal of small amounts of tissue from your body to test for disease.

blood stem cell
A blood-forming cell from which all other types of blood cells are formed. Also called hematopoietic stem cell.

body surface area
The total surface area of the human body, calculated using weight and height.

bone marrow
The sponge-like tissue in the center of most bones where blood cells are formed.

chemotherapy
Drugs that kill fast-growing cells, including normal cells and cancer cells.

chronic
An illness that keeps coming back or lasts a long time.

clinical trial
A study of how safe and helpful tests and treatments are for people.

complete blood count (CBC)
A lab test that measures the number of blood cells.

CT scan
A test that uses x-rays from many angles to make detailed pictures of the inside of the body.

contrast
A substance put into your body to make clearer pictures during imaging tests.

dermatologist
A health care provider who specializes in the diagnosis and treatment of skin diseases.

erythroderma
A severe inflammation of most of the body's skin surface. It can look like sunburn or large splotches.

hematopoietic cell transplant (HCT)
A type of treatment that destroys cells in the bone marrow and then replaces them with new, healthy blood-forming cells from another person. Also called stem cell transplant or bone marrow transplant.

human leukocyte antigen
A cell protein by which your body knows its own cells from foreign cells.

imaging test
A test that makes pictures (images) of the insides of the body.

immune system
The body's natural defense against infection and disease.

milliliter (mL)
A metric unit of volume equal to one thousandth of a liter.

MRI scan
A test that uses magnets and radio waves to make detailed pictures of the inside of the body.

palliative care
Special medical care for increasing quality of life and reducing pain and discomfort for people with serious, complex illnesses.

papule
A small, solid, raised bump on the skin that might look like a small pimple. Papules may be red, purple, brown, or pink.

patch
A flat, thin, pink or red skin lesion of any size.

pathologist
An expert in testing cells and tissue to find disease.

peripheral blood
Blood that circulates throughout the body.

phototherapy
A therapy that uses different ultraviolet (UV) light wavelengths to treat skin lesions or tumors.

plaque
A raised or hardened skin lesion of any size.

platelet
A type of blood cell that helps control bleeding. Also called a thrombocyte.

pruritus
An itchy feeling that makes you want to scratch your skin.

radiation oncologist
A health care provider who's an expert in treating cancer with radiation.

radiation therapy
A treatment that uses high-energy rays or related approaches to kill cancer cells.

radiologist
A health care provider who is an expert in imaging tests.

red blood cell
A type of blood cell that carries oxygen from the lungs to the rest of the body. Also called an erythrocyte.

scale
When the outer layer of skin peels away in large pieces.

side effect
An unhealthy or unpleasant physical or emotional response to treatment.

skin-directed therapy
Treatment focused on the skin. Includes topical therapy, local radiation, and phototherapy.

steroid-refractory disease
A condition where graft-versus host disease (GVHD) stops responding to or worsens on steroid treatment.

supportive care
Health care that includes symptom relief but not cancer treatment. Also called palliative care.

systemic therapy
Treatment that works throughout the body.

targeted therapy
A drug treatment that targets and attacks specific cancer cells.

ulcer
A break in the skin that exposes underlying tissue.

white blood cell
A type of blood cell that helps fight infections in the body. Also called a leukocyte.

NCCN Contributors

This patient guide is based on the NCCN Clinical Practice Guidelines in Oncology (NCCN Guidelines®) for Hematopoietic Cell Transplantation, Version 3.2025. It was adapted, reviewed, and published with help from the following people:

Dorothy A. Shead, MS
Senior Director
Patient Information Operations

Tim Rinehart, MS
Medical Writer

Lisa Diehl
Production Layout Artist

The NCCN Clinical Practice Guidelines in Oncology (NCCN Guidelines®) for Hematopoietic Cell Transplantation, Version 3.2025 were developed by the following NCCN Panel Members:

Alison W. Loren, MD, MSCE/Chair
Abramson Cancer Center
at the University of Pennsylvania

Marco Mielcarek, MD, PhD/
Vice-Chair
Fred Hutchinson Cancer Center

Mathew Angelos, MD, PhD
University of Colorado Cancer Center

Javier Bolaños-Meade, MD
Johns Hopkins Kimmel Cancer Center

Jonathan Brammer, MD
The Ohio State University Comprehensive Cancer Center - James Cancer Hospital and Solove Research Institute

*Meredith Cowden, MA
Meredith A. Cowden Foundation

Antonio Di Stasi, MD
O'Neal Comprehensive
Cancer Center at UAB

Areej El-Jawahri, MD
Mass General Cancer Center

Hany Elmariah, MD, MS
Moffitt Cancer Center

Krishna Gundabolu, MBBS, MS
Fred & Pamela Buffett Cancer Center

Jonathan Gutman, MD
University of Colorado Cancer Center

Vincent Ho, MD
Dana-Farber/Brigham and
Women's Cancer Center

Rasmus T. Hoeg, MD
UC Davis Comprehensive Cancer Center

Mitchell Horwitz, MD
Duke Cancer Institute

Omer Jamy, MD
O'Neal Comprehensive
Cancer Center at UAB

Adetola Kassim, MD, MS
Vanderbilt-Ingram Cancer Center

*Mohamed Kharfan Dabaja, MD
Mayo Clinic Comprehensive Cancer Center

Lauren Lee, MD
Huntsman Cancer Institute at the University of Utah

Aaron Logan, MD, PhD, MPhil
UCSF Helen Diller Family
Comprehensive Cancer Center

Christina Luszcak, PharmD, BCOP
Case Comprehensive Cancer Center/
University Hospitals Seidman Cancer Center
and Cleveland Clinic Taussig Cancer Institute

John M. Magenau, MD
University of Michigan Rogel Cancer Center

Thomas G. Martin, MD
UCSF Helen Diller Family
Comprehensive Cancer Center

Varun Mittal, MD
Indiana University Melvin and Bren Simon
Comprehensive Cancer Center

Jonathan Moreira, MD
Robert H. Lurie Comprehensive Cancer
Center of Northwestern University

Lori Muffly, MD
Stanford Cancer Institute

*Ryotaro Nakamura, MD
City of Hope National Medical Center

Mariam Nawas, MD
The UChicago Medicine
Comprehensive Cancer Center

Yago Nieto, MD, PhD
The University of Texas
MD Anderson Cancer Center

Cameron Ninos, PharmD
University of Wisconsin
Carbone Cancer Center

Caspian Oliai, MD
UCLA Jonsson
Comprehensive Cancer Center

Genovefa Papanicolaou, MD
Memorial Sloan Kettering Cancer Center

*Joseph Pidala, MD, PhD
Moffitt Cancer Center

Brion Randolph, MD
St. Jude Children's
Research Hospital/
The University of Tennessee
Health Science Center

Grant Schofield, MD, MSc
Roswell Park Comprehensive Cancer Center

Mark A. Schroeder, MD
Siteman Cancer Center at Barnes-
Jewish Hospital and Washington
University School of Medicine

Jeffrey Tessier, MD
UT Southwestern Simmons
Comprehensive Cancer Center

Jeffrey Topal, MD
Yale Cancer Center/Smilow Cancer Hospital

Dimitrios Tzachanis MD, PhD
UC San Diego Moores Cancer Center

Asya Nina Varshavsky-Yanovsky,
MD, PhD
Fox Chase Cancer Center

NCCN

Frankie Jones
Guidelines Coordinator

Katie Stehman, MMS, PA-C
Oncology Scientist/Senior Medical Writer

* Reviewed this patient guide. For disclosures, visit NCCN.org/disclosures.

NCCN Cancer Centers

For contact information visit NCCN.org/cancercenters.

Abramson Cancer Center
at the University of Pennsylvania
Philadelphia, Pennsylvania

Case Comprehensive Cancer Center/
University Hospitals Seidman Cancer Center and
Cleveland Clinic Taussig Cancer Institute
Cleveland, Ohio

City of Hope National Medical Center
Duarte, California

Dana-Farber/Brigham and Women's Cancer Center |
Mass General Cancer Center
Boston, Massachusetts

Duke Cancer Institute
Durham, North Carolina

Fox Chase Cancer Center
Philadelphia, Pennsylvania

Fred & Pamela Buffett Cancer Center
Omaha, Nebraska

Fred Hutchinson Cancer Center
Seattle, Washington

Huntsman Cancer Institute at the University of Utah
Salt Lake City, Utah

Indiana University Melvin and Bren Simon
Comprehensive Cancer Center
Indianapolis, Indiana

Johns Hopkins Kimmel Cancer Center
Baltimore, Maryland

Mayo Clinic Comprehensive Cancer Center
Phoenix/Scottsdale, Arizona
Jacksonville, Florida
Rochester, Minnesota

Memorial Sloan Kettering Cancer Center
New York, New York

Moffitt Cancer Center
Tampa, Florida

O'Neal Comprehensive Cancer Center at UAB
Birmingham, Alabama

Robert H. Lurie Comprehensive Cancer Center
of Northwestern University
Chicago, Illinois

Roswell Park Comprehensive Cancer Center
Buffalo, New York

Siteman Cancer Center at Barnes-Jewish Hospital
and Washington University School of Medicine
St. Louis, Missouri

St. Jude Children's Research Hospital/
The University of Tennessee Health Science Center
Memphis, Tennessee

Stanford Cancer Institute
Stanford, California

The Ohio State University Comprehensive Cancer Center -
James Cancer Hospital and Solove Research Institute
Columbus, Ohio

The UChicago Medicine Comprehensive Cancer Center
Chicago, Illinois

The University of Texas MD Anderson Cancer Center
Houston, Texas

UC Davis Comprehensive Cancer Center
Sacramento, California

UC San Diego Moores Cancer Center
La Jolla, California

UCLA Jonsson Comprehensive Cancer Center
Los Angeles, California

UCSF Helen Diller Family Comprehensive Cancer Center
San Francisco, California

University of Colorado Cancer Center
Aurora, Colorado

University of Michigan Rogel Cancer Center
Ann Arbor, Michigan

University of Wisconsin Carbone Cancer Center
Madison, Wisconsin

UT Southwestern Simmons
Comprehensive Cancer Center
Dallas, Texas

Vanderbilt-Ingram Cancer Center
Nashville, Tennessee

Yale Cancer Center/Smilow Cancer Hospital
New Haven, Connecticut

Notes

Index

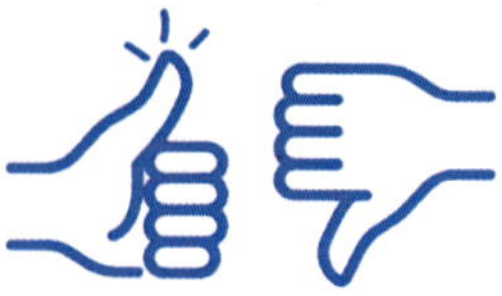

Let us know what you think!

Please take a moment to complete an online survey about the NCCN Guidelines for Patients.
NCCN.org/patients/response

Made in United States
North Haven, CT
05 November 2026

21765510R00027